Principles of
Laboratory Instruments

Principles of Laboratory Instruments

Larry E. Schoeff, M.S., MT (ASCP)
Director and Associate Professor
Medical Technology Program
Department of Pathology
University of Utah School of Medicine

Education Director
Associated Regional and University Pathologists, Inc. (ARUP)
Salt Lake City, Utah

Robert H. Williams, Ph.D., MT (ASCP)
Director, Section of General Chemistry/Toxicology
University of Illinois Hospital
Division of Clinical Pathology
Department of Pathology, College of Medicine
University of Illinois at Chicago
Chicago, Illinois

*with **315** illustrations*

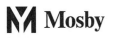 Mosby

St. Louis Baltimore Boston Chicago London Philadelphia Sydney Toronto

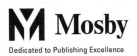

Dedicated to Publishing Excellence

Editor: Stephanie Manning
Assistant Editor: Jane Petrash
Project Manager: John A. Rogers
Senior Production Editor: Shauna Burnett Sticht
Designer: David Zielinski

Printed in the United States of America

Mosby–Year Book, Inc.
11830 Westline Industrial Drive
St. Louis, Missouri 63146

Library of Congress Cataloging in Publication Data
Principles of laboratory instruments / [edited by] Larry E. Schoeff,
Robert H. Williams.
    p. cm.
   Includes bibliographical references and index.
   ISBN 0-8016-7489-1
   1. Diagnosis, Laboratory—Instruments. 2. Medical laboratories
—Instruments. I. Schoeff, Larry E. II. Williams, Robert H.
(Robert Henry),
   [DNLM: 1. Equipment and Supplies. 2. Laboratories.
3. Technology, Medical—instrumentation. W 26 P957]
RB36.2.P75 1992
610′.28—dc20
DNLM/DLC
for Library of Congress   92-49752
                              CIP

93 94 95 96 97 UG/MY 9 8 7 6 5 4 3 2 1

Contributors

Lemuel Bowie, Ph.D., DABCC
Clinical Chemistry Laboratory
Evanston Hospital
Evanston, Illinois

John M. Brewer, Ph.D.
Department of Biochemistry
University of Georgia
Athens, Georgia

I-Wen Chen, Ph.D.
Department of Radiobiology Laboratory
University of Cincinnati Medical Center
Cincinnati, Ohio

Mary Ann Dotson, MT (ASCP), CLS (NCA)
Duke University Medical Center
Durham, North Carolina

David Hage, Ph.D.
University of Nebraska
Lincoln, Nebraska

Debra Hoppensteadt, MS, MT (ASCP)
Department of Pathology
Loyola University Medical Center
Maywood, Illinois

Barbara Lewis, MS, SM (ASCP)
Management and Microbiology Consultant
Batavia, Illinois

Sherwood C. Lewis, Ph.D., DABCC
Department of Pathology and Laboratory
    Medicine
St. Francis Hospital and Medical Center
Hartford, Connecticut
Department of Laboratory Medicine
University of Connecticut School of Medicine
Farmington, Connecticut

Jack Maggiore, MS, MT (ASCP)
University of Illinois Hospital
Chicago, Illinois

Andrew Maturen, Ph.D., DABCC, MT (ASCP)
OCLS Clinical Chemistry
Rush Presbyterian St. Luke's Medical Center
Chicago, Illinois

Anthony O. Okorodudu, Ph.D., DABCC
Clinical Chemistry Division
Department of Pathology
University of Texas Medical Branch
Galveston, Texas

Marguerite Quale, M.S., MT (ASCP)
Ravenswood Hospital Medical Center
Chicago, Illinois

Kathy Ristow, MT (ASCP)
Clinical Microbiology Laboratory
University of Illinois Hospital
Chicago, Illinois

Jeanine Walenga, Ph.D., MT (ASCP)
Department of Pathology
Loyola University Medical Center
Maywood, Illinois

Robert Webster, Ph.D., DABCC
OCLS Clinical Chemistry
Rush Presbyterian St. Luke's Medical Center
Chicago, Illinois

Preface

The intended audience for **Principles of Laboratory Instruments** includes all clinical laboratorians who expect to operate laboratory instruments. In addition to students of clinical laboratory science, this may include pathology residents, medical students, and graduate students in the medical sciences. Much of the information provided in this text should also be invaluable to clinical chemists, pathologists, supervisory personnel in the clinical laboratory sciences, and others who may have a vested interest in laboratory medicine, such as instrument manufacturers.

No field in medicine has expanded as rapidly as laboratory medicine, especially in the area of laboratory automation. Understanding how an instrument operates is difficult because of the great variation in the complexity of instrumentation that exists, especially in today's marketplace where instrumentation has become highly computerized. It is paramount that individuals working in this field have a basic understanding of the function of electronic components and units used in the manufacturing of instruments, those principles applied to instruments that are inherent in their operation, and the concept of instrument subsystems and how they are integrated to form a functioning unit. In addition they should be knowledgeable about the instruments that are currently available in the marketplace, have a working knowledge of their unique characteristics, and be aware of their applications to patient testing in the clinical laboratory.

It is hoped that teaching the basic principles and theory of instrumental analysis as applied to the field of laboratory medicine will provide a working knowledge for instrument selection; an effective means of instruction for operators to make proper judgments during the operation of an instrument and to recognize the limitations, advantages, and disadvantages of each; a means of identifying instrumental problems; and common approaches to troubleshooting some of the problems that cause an instrument to malfunction.

The purpose of this text is twofold: to provide a foundation of knowledge in basic electronics and principles of instrumentation, and to apply the theoretic principles of electronics and instrumentation to the automated systems that are currently available in the marketplace. To accomplish these goals the text has been organized into three sections: **Basic Electricity and Electronic Components, Principles of Instrumentation, and Automation in the Clinical Laboratory.** The section on Basic Electricity and Electronic Components covers basic and intermediate principles of electronics and serves as a background for subsequent sections. The section on Principles of Instrumentation covers basic principles that are applied to instrumental analysis and addresses specific instruments that employ that particular mode of analysis. The last section, Automation in the Clinical Laboratory, contains information pertaining to automation in general and is divided according to subspecialty, describing in detail the principles of operation and unique features for many of the major instruments that are currently used in the clinical laboratory.

With the rapid advances and changes in instrumentation technology it is difficult for a book of this nature to remain up-to-date. What is "cutting edge" technology today, seen as concepts on design tables and prototypes in research and development laboratories, can become reality in clinical laboratories in a matter of months. Such "hot" topics as front-end automation (robotics); in vivo, noninvasive mobile analyzers; spectral mapping for simultaneous, multiple chemistries; artificial intelligence in analyzers; enhanced system integration and miniaturization; and other new concepts will likely appear in the clinical laboratory in the not too distant future. We hope to include these topics in the next edition of **Principles of Laboratory Instruments.**

Larry E. Schoeff
Robert H. Williams

Table of Contents

Principles of
Laboratory Instruments